Table of Content

Introduction

Grilled Pineapple

   Tomato Salmon

   Noodle Stir Fry with Shrimp

   Avocado Toast with Kale

   Grilled Salmon with Foil

   Chicken & Bell Pepper Stir Fry

   Chinese Ramen Noodle

   Baked Squash Blossom

   Pumpkin Pie Chocolate Chip Yogurt

   Beef Noodle Stir Fry

   Sweet and Spicy Salmon

   Fried Apple

   Simple Stir Fry Noodle

   Spinach with Sesame Oil

   Kiwi and Mango Yogurt

   Kale and Spinach Smoothie

   Vietnamese Rice Noodle

   Spinach and Cheese Cups

   Baked Garlic Chicken

   Spinach and Kiwi Smoothie

   Asian Pineapple Chicken Stir Fry

Raspberry, Strawberry and Blueberry Smoothie

Pea Chicken Stir Fry

Beet, Raspberry, Strawberry and Mango Smoothie

Miso Honey Chicken

Peach and Mango Smoothie

Simple and Quick Avocado Smoothie

Minute Thai Chicken Stir Fry

Avocado Yogurt

Chicken Noodle and Ginger Sauce

Conclusion

Introduction

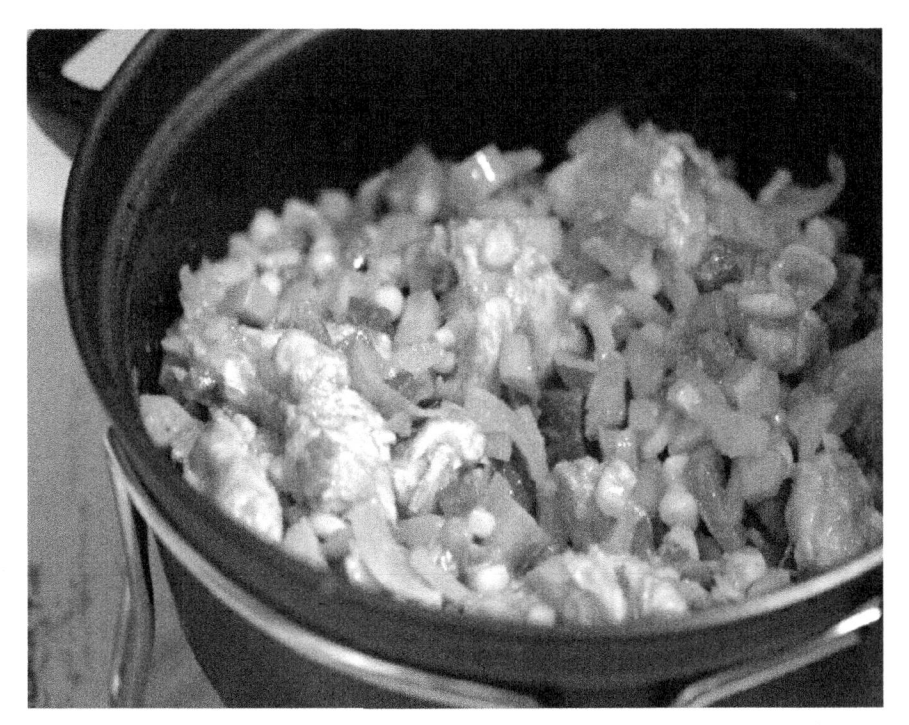

Let's begin this with an ugly truth I have learnt the hard way in my life: the ability to cook luxurious meals is not genetically inherited. The fact that your grandmother or your mother is a seasoned cook, does not necessarily mean that you will also be a good cook. Just like all skills in life, you will have to spend time in practice to improve your techniques. Most persons prefer quick and simple recipes that leave a smile on your face.

If your lifestyle is a busy one or the little angel in your tummy keeps you on your toes, or you are simply new to cooking, Hassle Free Pregnancy Cookbook will relieve you of your fears and increase the fun factor as you experiment with different flavors. The recipes in this book are simple and as you become a bit more experienced you can tweak to suit your preferred taste. This book will work wonders for you if you lead a busy lifestyle.

The recipes in this book are made from readily available ingredients or less and most can be served in 30 minutes or a little less, some of them can be done in a slow cooker while you relax. You can also pre - prepare when you have some time on your hands and freeze for reheating later.

Hassle Free Pregnancy Cookbook's goal is teaching you how to prepare simple delicious meals without having you spending long hours on your feet in the kitchen. The goal of this book is to show you how easy it is to make a delicious dinner without spending hours in the kitchen. Very important too, the biggest focus is using fresh ingredients as often as possible and keeping processed foods at a minimum to give you a healthy diet for a healthy baby.

Grilled Pineapple

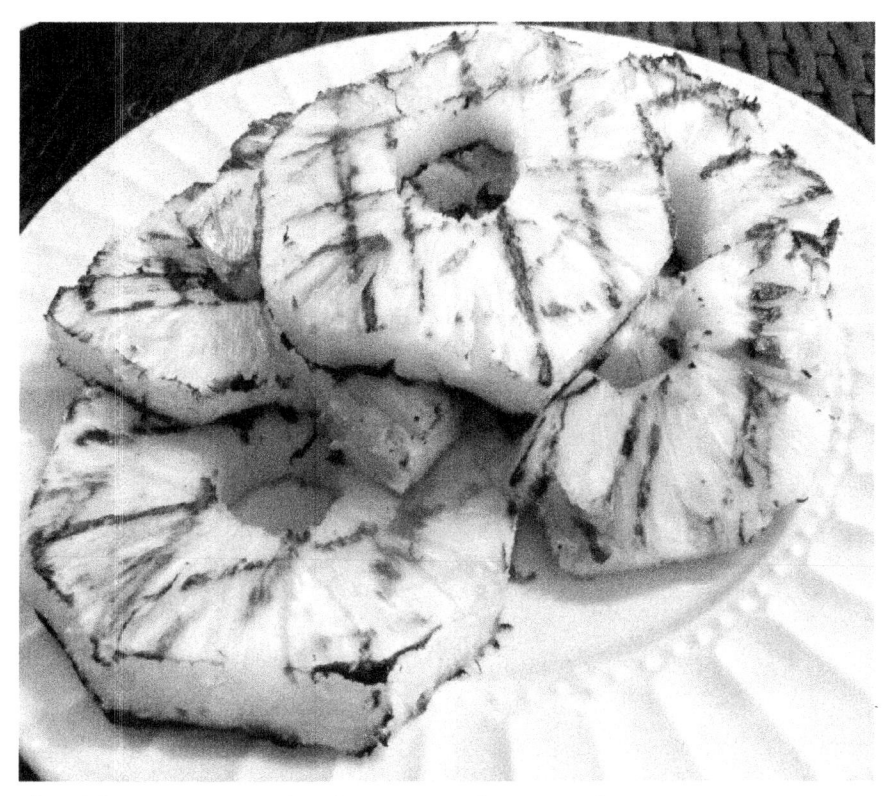

This delicious recipe makes for a tasty and easy snack.

Serves: 2

Time: 30 minutes

Ingredients:

- Cilantro (chopped) – ¼ cup
- Whole pineapple (cut into spears) – 1
- Olive oil – 3 tablespoons
- Red onion – ½ cup
- Pepper (chopped) – 1
- Lime juice – 2 tablespoons

Directions:

1. Preheat your grill over high medium heat.

2. Place the pineapple and grill for 5 – 10 minutes. Then remove from the grill.

3. Mix all the ingredients together, gently toss to coat.

4. Keep it in refrigerator.

Tomato Salmon

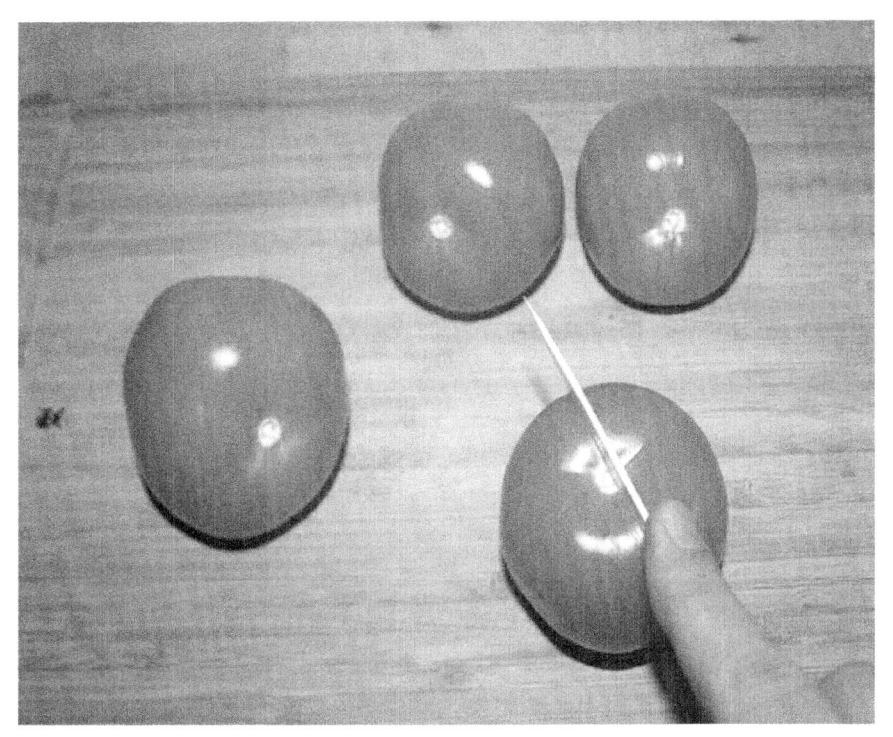

This salmon recipe provides the perfect level of acidity to help combat those nausea filled days.

Serves: 2

Time: 30 minutes

Ingredients:

- Salmon fillet – 2
- Grape tomato (cut into halve) – 1 cup
- Parchment paper – 2 (18-inche long pieces)
- Red onion (thin slices) – 4
- Basil leave – 5
- Olive oil – 1 tablespoon
- Balsamic vinegar – 1 tablespoon
- Salt – 1 teaspoon
- Pepper – 1 teaspoon

Directions:

1. Place a parchment paper on a baking sheet, spray with a bit cooking oil.

2. Place salmon fillets on the baking sheet, then place grape tomatoes, onions and basil around the salmon and season all the ingredients with salt and pepper.

3. Next is season all the ingredients with 1 tablespoon of olive oil and 1 tablespoon of Balsamic vinegar.

4. Wrap salmon and veggies by folding it over itself, then bake the salmon at 400 degrees for 10 – 15 minutes.

5. Remove from the oven, open and enjoy.

Noodle Stir Fry with Shrimp

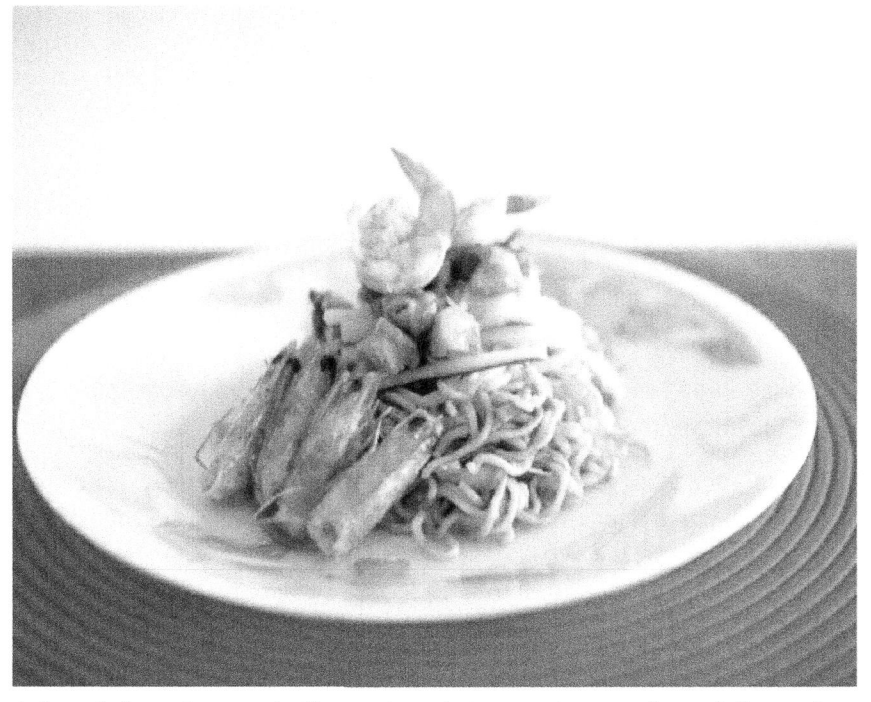

A lot of the spices typically used in Asian cuisine can be red flags when pregnant for nausea, however when used in the perfect ratio those same spices can act as a delicious amplifier for your dish. Here is one such recipe.

Serves: 6

Time: 30 minutes

Ingredients:

- Noodle (linguini) – 12 ounces
- Shrimp (peeled and deveined with tails removed) – 2 pounds
- Soy sauce – ½ cup
- Cornstarch – 8 teaspoons
- Fresh ginger (grated) – ½ tablespoon
- Garlic (minced) – 6 cloves
- Sesame oil – 4 teaspoons
- Carrot (shredded) – 2 cups
- Cabbage (thin slices) – 2 cups

- Chicken broth – ½ cup
- Green onion (cut into strips) – 7

Directions:

1. Let shrimp marinated in the mixture of soy sauce, garlic, ginger and cornstarch for 10 minutes.

2. Meanwhile, cook the noodle in a large pot for 1 minute. (10 minutes to wait for water being boiled and 1 minutes to cook the noodle).

3. Remove shrimp and drain. Set a half of your sesame oil to get hot in a wok.

4. Add the shrimp and stir fry for 3 minutes. When the shrimps are pink, it is alright to remove from the wok.

5. Add in your other half of sesame oil to the same wok, then add carrot, cabbage and stir fry for 2 minutes. Pour the chicken broth and the reserve marinade to the wok.

6. When the mixture of carrot, cabbage and chicken broth is cooked through, return the cooked shrimps to the wok and cook.

7. Pour the mixture of cooked shrimps in chicken broth to the cooked noodle. Mix them well, top with green onions and serve.

Avocado Toast with Kale

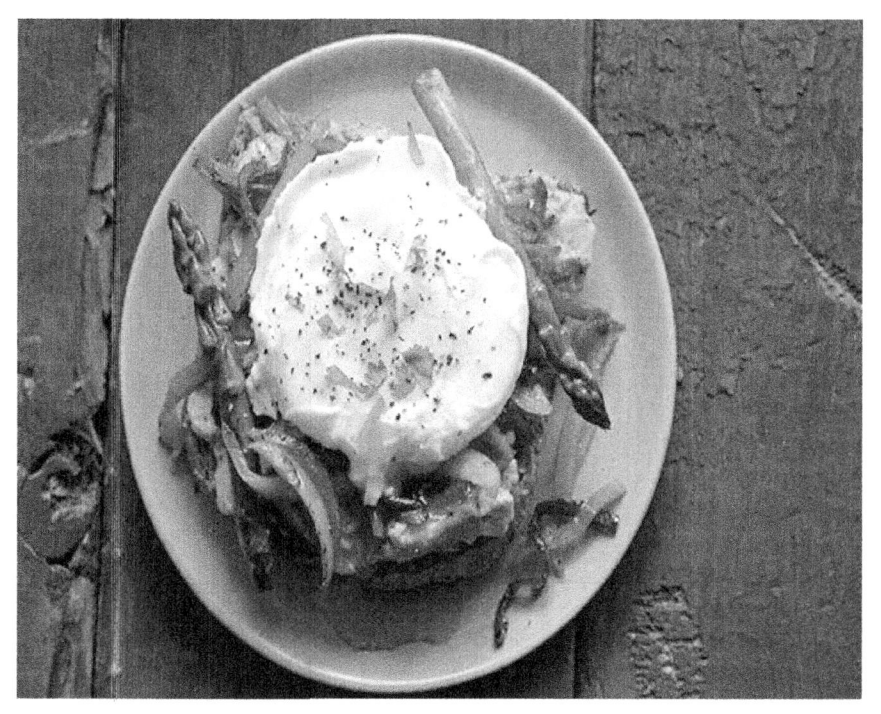

For a simple breakfast that can be whipped up in minutes, this recipe will become your best bet.

Serves: 2

Time: 30 minutes

Ingredients:

- Kale – 1 cup
- Lemon – ½
- Avocado – 4 ounces
- Olive oil – 1 teaspoon
- Bread – 4 slices
- Cumin – 1/8 teaspoon
- Radish (sliced) – 4 slices
- Chia seeds – 1 teaspoon
- Salt and pepper

Directions:

1. In a bowl, add kale, olive oil, lemon juice and a little salt and mix them well.

2. Halve the avocado. Cut into slices one of them. And smash the other. Season the smash avocado with a little salt, pepper and lemon juice.

3. Toast the slices of bread

4. Spread the smashed avocado on the toasted bread slices, then place slices of avocado on top and sprinkle a little salt, pepper and cumin.

5. Place the mixture of kale, radish and chia seeds on top of bread. And serve.

Grilled Salmon with Foil

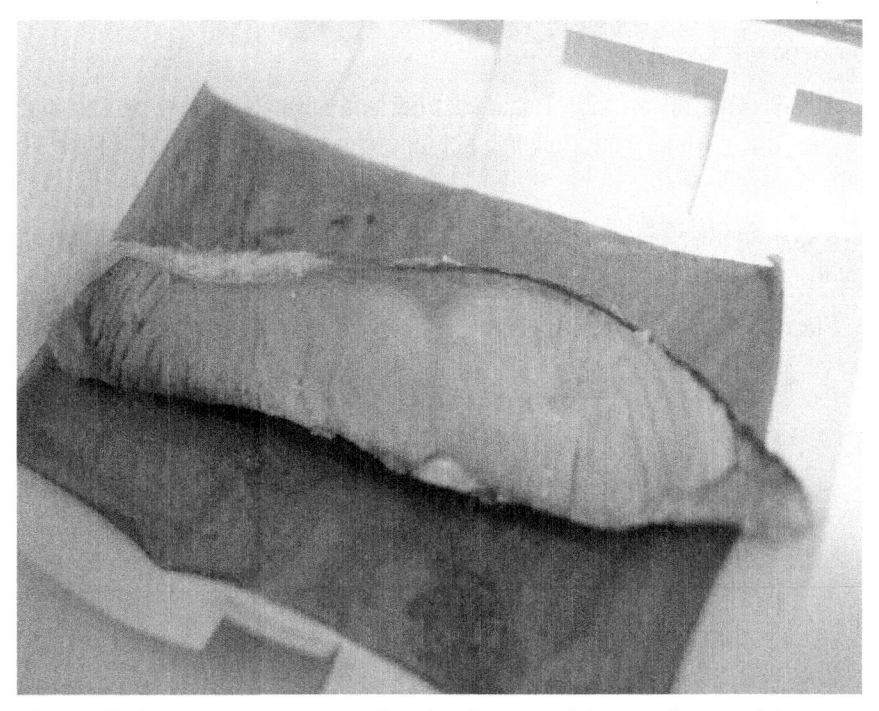

This Grilled Salmon recipe is perfect for those tired days and super delicious.

Serves: 2

Time: 15 minutes

Ingredients:

- Boneless salmon fillet – 2 (3/4 inch thick each)
- Large piece of aluminum foil – 2
- White wine – ¼ cup
- Lemon (cut into thin slices) – 1
- Lemon juice – 3 tablespoons
- Olive oil – 3 tablespoons
- Kosher salt – ½ teaspoon
- Freshly ground black pepper – ½ teaspoon
- Caper – 1 tablespoon

Directions:

1. Heat your grill to 450 degrees.

2. Carefully line a baking sheet with foil, then place the salmon, skin side down on the baking sheet.

3. Brush olive oil on top of salmon fillet and sprinkle with a bit salt and pepper, then white wine, lemon juice and capers, finally, place a slice of lemon on top.

4. Place another piece of foil over the salmon, let salmon fillets wrapped tightly in foil.

5. Place the salmon on grill and cook for 10 - 20 minutes, then take it out and serve.

Chicken & Bell Pepper Stir Fry

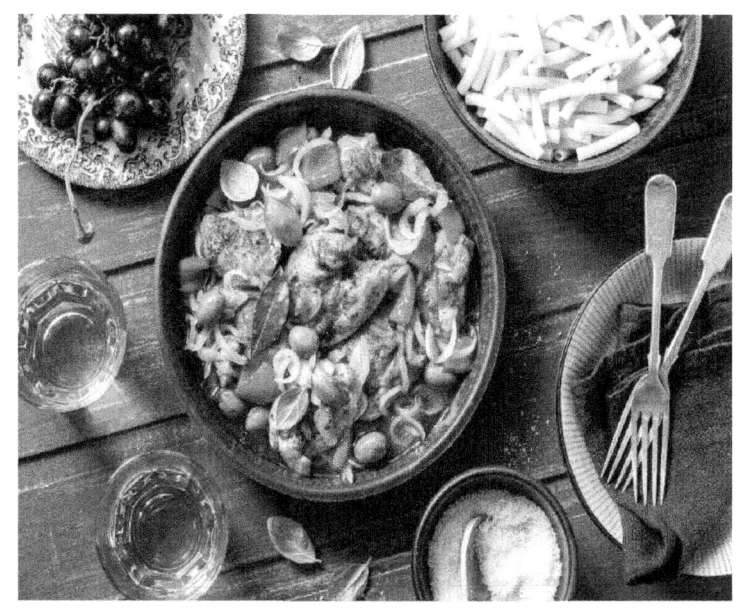

This tasty stir-fry is easy whip up and yields enough for a small family.

Serves: 2 - 3

Time: 30 minutes

Ingredients:

- Boneless Chicken (cut into bite-size pieces) – 8 ounces
- Bell pepper (cut into bite-size pieces) – 2
- Onion 1 large (thinly sliced)
- Fish sauce – 2 tablespoons
- Oyster sauce – 1 tablespoon
- Sugar – 1 teaspoon
- Canola – 2 tablespoons
- Garlic (chopped) – 2 cloves
- Ginger (chopped) – 2 tablespoons
- Green onion (cut into 1-inch pieces) – 2

Directions:

1. Mix fish sauce, oyster sauce and sugar well together in a bowl.

2. Set your oil on in a wok to get hot on high heat. Add in your garlic and allow to cook for a minute, before adding the chicken and ginger, stir and cook for 5 minutes.

3. Add the bell pepper, green onions, onions, stir and cook for 3 minutes,

4. Then add the mixture of sauce and cook for 3 minutes to let the chicken is fully cooked.

5. Remove the wok from heat. And your dish is ready to serve with rice. Enjoy!

Chinese Ramen Noodle

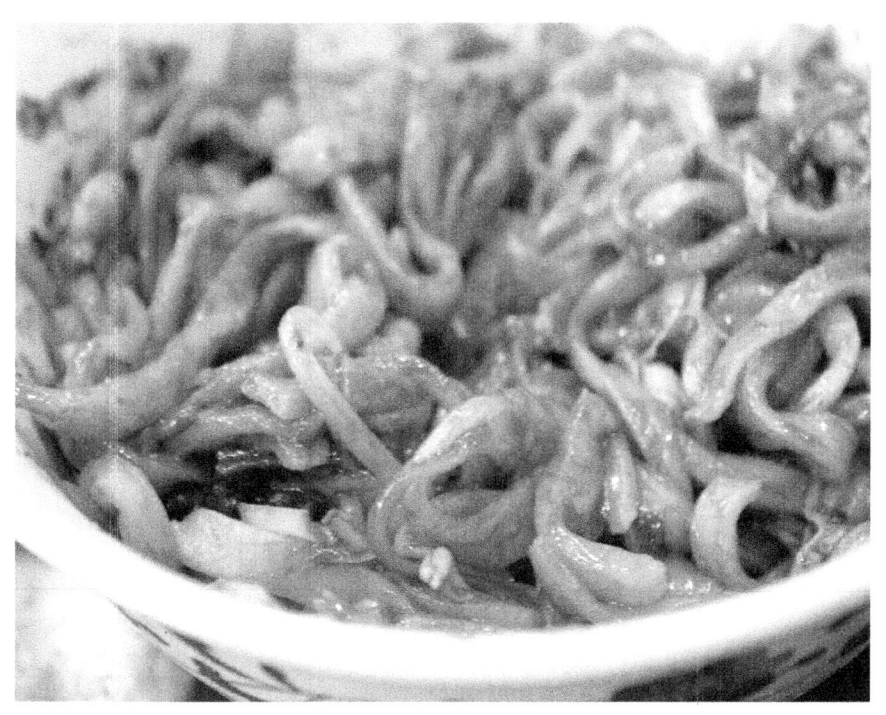

Ramen Noodles, despite popular belief, is in no way only for college students. This recipe teaches you how to come up with a delicious, sophisticated meal.

Serves: 4

Time: 30 minutes

Ingredients:

- Ramen Noodles – 2 packages
- Chicken stock – ½ cup
- Oyster sauce – 1/3 cup
- Cauliflower (cut into smaller pieces) – ½ of big floret
- Baby corn – 125 g
- Ground white pepper – ½ teaspoon
- Corn flour – 1 teaspoon
- Onion (thin slices) – 2
- Oil – 2 tablespoons

- Garlic (chopped) – 2 cloves
- Ginger (chopped) – 2cm piece

Directions:

1. Set your oil on in a wok to get hot, add garlic, onion and ginger to the wok, stir fry for 1 minute and add cauliflower and baby corn, continue to cook for 3 minutes.

2. Add oyster sauce and pepper, stir fry for 2 minutes.

3. Mix corn flour with chicken stock together in a bowl. Add this mixture to the wok, stir to mix it well with vegetable.

4. When the mixture begins to thicken, add noodle and stir for 3 minutes.

5. Remove the wok and place the noodle on a plate.

Baked Squash Blossom

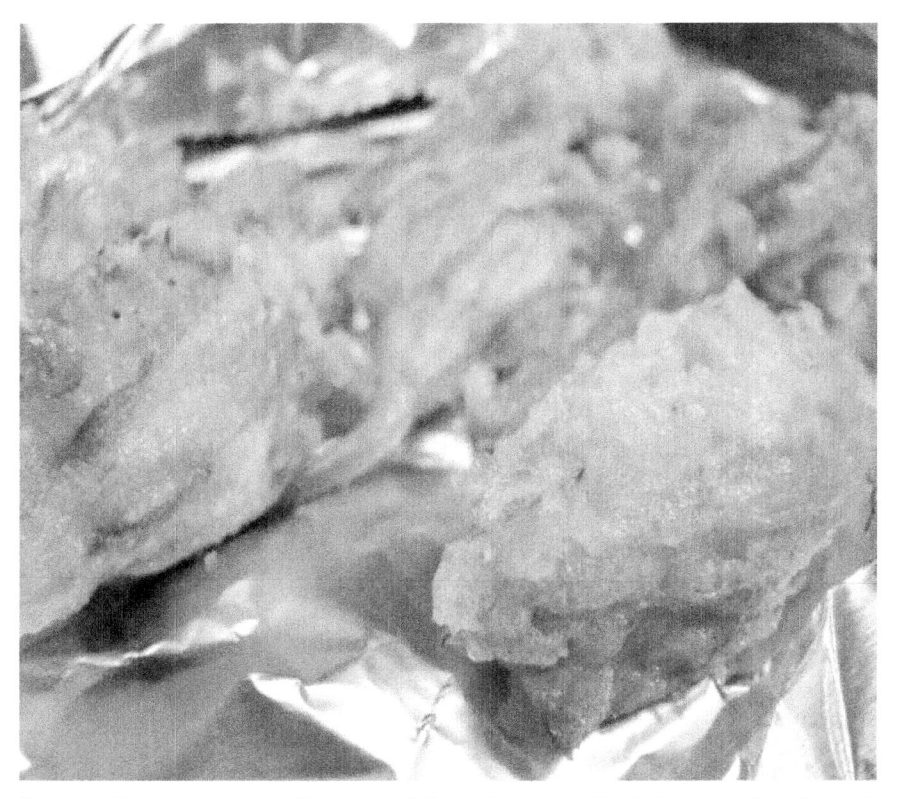

Squash blossoms are easily accessible and extremely delicious when baked. Don't take my word for it, try it for yourself.

Serves: 2

Time: 30 minutes

Ingredients:

- Squash blossom – 12
- Ricotta – 1 cup
- Egg (divided) – 3
- Parsley – 1/3 cup
- Breadcrumb – ¾ cup
- Salt – 1 teaspoon

Directions:

1. Preheat the oven to 400 degrees.

2. Combine 1 egg, ricotta, parsley and a little salt well together. Mix them well.

3. Crack the remaining eggs and beat them well in a bowl.

4. Filling the squash blossoms with the mixture of ricotta and egg.

5. Then dip the stuffed squash blossoms in egg, breadcrumbs, then place them on baking sheet lined with parchment paper, then bake for 10 minutes. Enjoy!

Pumpkin Pie Chocolate Chip Yogurt

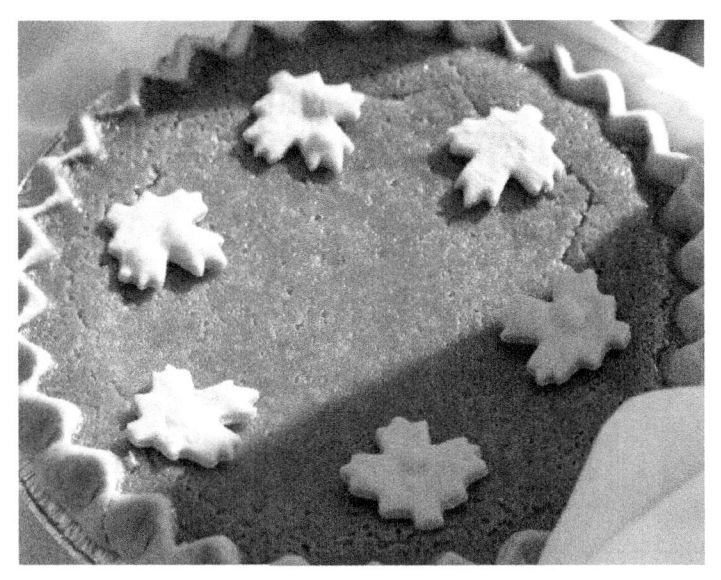

For a quick ease to your ever-growing sweet tooth then this yogurt has got you covered.

Serves: 1

Time: 5 minutes

Ingredients:

- Pumpkin pie yogurt- ½ cup
- Chocolate Chex™ cereal (crushed) – ¼ cup
- Semisweet chocolate chip – 2 teaspoons
- Frozen whipped cream – 2 tablespoons

Directions:

1. Add half of yogurt in the bottom of glass, then add cereal and chocolate chip, pour the remaining yogurt and top with frozen whipped cream.

2. Serve.

Beef Noodle Stir Fry

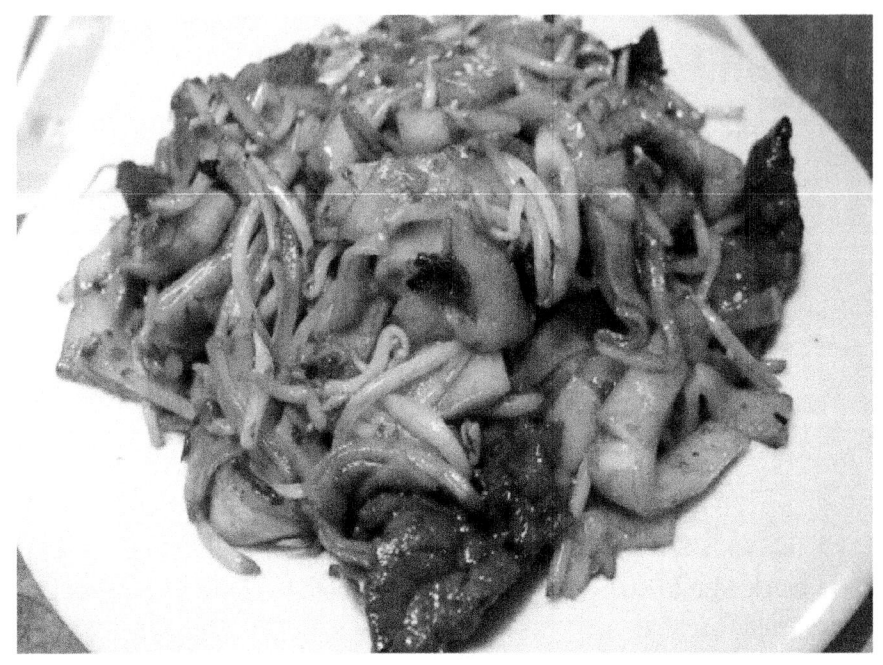

Stir fried dishes are extremely easy pull off, making them perfect for any busy night.

Serves: 2

Time: 25 minutes

Ingredients:

- Beef (thin slices) – 1 pound
- Noodle – 2 packages
- Carrot (thin slices) – 1
- Red pepper (thin slices) – 1
- Broccoli (cooked and cut into small pieces) – 1 floret
- Fish sauce – 3 tablespoons
- Garlic (minced) – 1 clove
- Onion (chopped) - 1
- Salt – ½ teaspoon
- Pepper – ¼ teaspoon

Directions:

1. Add the water to a pot, bring to a boil, add the noodle to the pot and cook (about a minute), remove and drain.

2. With the remaining water, cook the broccoli for 3 minutes.

3. After that, heat the oil in a pan, add the minced garlic, chopped onion and stir for 30 seconds until fragrant.

4. Then add the beef to the pan stir for 3 minutes, then add broccoli, carrot, red pepper and fish sauce, salt and pepper, stir and cook for another 5 minutes to make sure all ingredients are tender.

5. Serve.

Sweet and Spicy Salmon

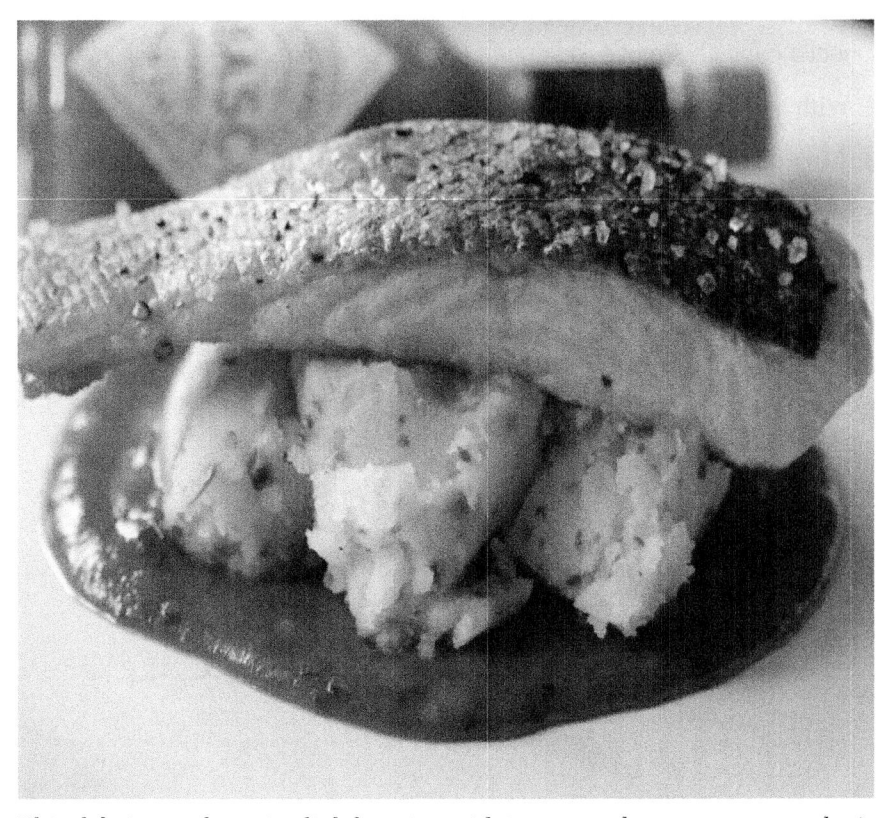

This delicious salmon is slightly spicy with just enough sweetness to make it delicious.

Serves: 2

Time: 20 minutes

Ingredients:

- Boneless salmon fillet – 2 (½ lb. each)
- Lemon juice – ½ teaspoon
- Cajun seasoning – 1 tablespoon
- Peach jam – 1 tablespoon
- Cooking oil – 2 teaspoons
- Brown sugar – 1 teaspoon

Directions:

1. Mix sugar with Cajun seasoning well together in a bowl. Season the salmon fillets with the mixture of Cajun evenly.

2. Heat oil in a non-stick pan over medium heat, then place the salmon on the pan, allow to cook for 5 minutes each side.

3. Mix peach jam with lemon juice, then add this mixture to hot pan, let it coat evenly the fillets, cook until the sauce gets thicken.

4. Remove fish from pan, you can eat salmon alone or pair it with any sauce. Enjoy!

Fried Apple

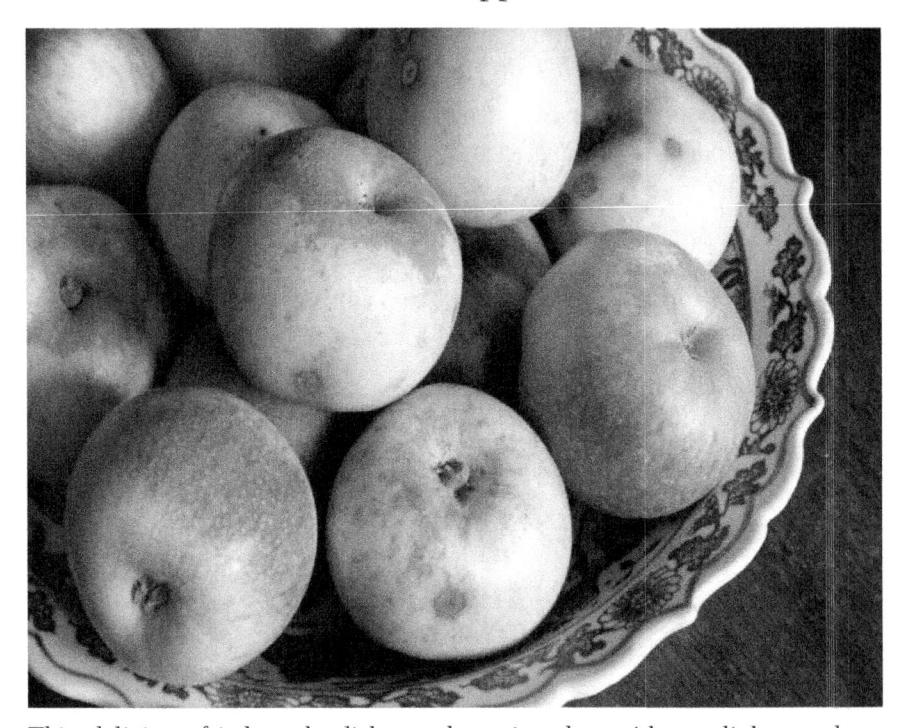

This delicious fried apple dish can be enjoyed as either a light snack or dessert.

Serves: 1

Time: 25 minutes

Ingredients:

- Apple (cut into cubes or thick slices) – 2, large
- Butter (chopped) – 4 tablespoons
- White sugar – 2 tablespoons
- Brown sugar – 2 tablespoons
- Lemon juice – ½
- Cinnamon – 1 teaspoon

Directions:

1. Heat the skillet and let the butter melted.

2. Add the apple, stir and add lemon juice into the skillet, cook until the apples are tender.

3. Add sugar and stir well to coat evenly the apples.

4. Add cinnamon to the apples, toss to coat.

5. Remove from heat. Serve.

Simple Stir Fry Noodle

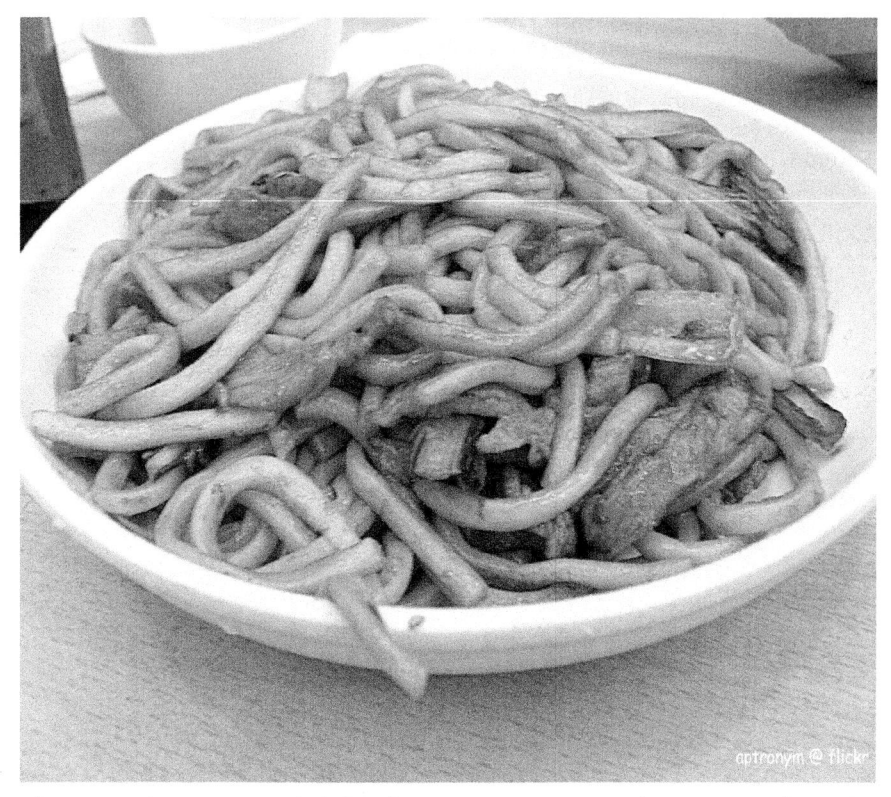

This tasty Asian inspired dish whips up in a matter of minutes and can be enjoyed at any time of the day.

Serves: 4

Time: 30 minutes

Ingredients:

- Steam fried Chinese noodle – 7 ounces
- Ginger – 6 slices
- Green onion (cut into 1-inch strips) – 2
- Oil – 3 tablespoons

For the sauce:

- Oyster sauce – 3 tablespoons

- Soya sauce – 2 tablespoons
- Sesame oil – 1 tablespoon

Directions:

1. Set your water on to boil, add in your noodles, and cook for 2 minutes, remove and drain.

2. Add oil to a pan. When it is heated, add ginger, and onion to the pan, stir fry until fragrant.

3. Add noodle, stir fry for 5 minutes.

4. Add the mixture of sauce, toss to coat.

5. Serve.

Spinach with Sesame Oil

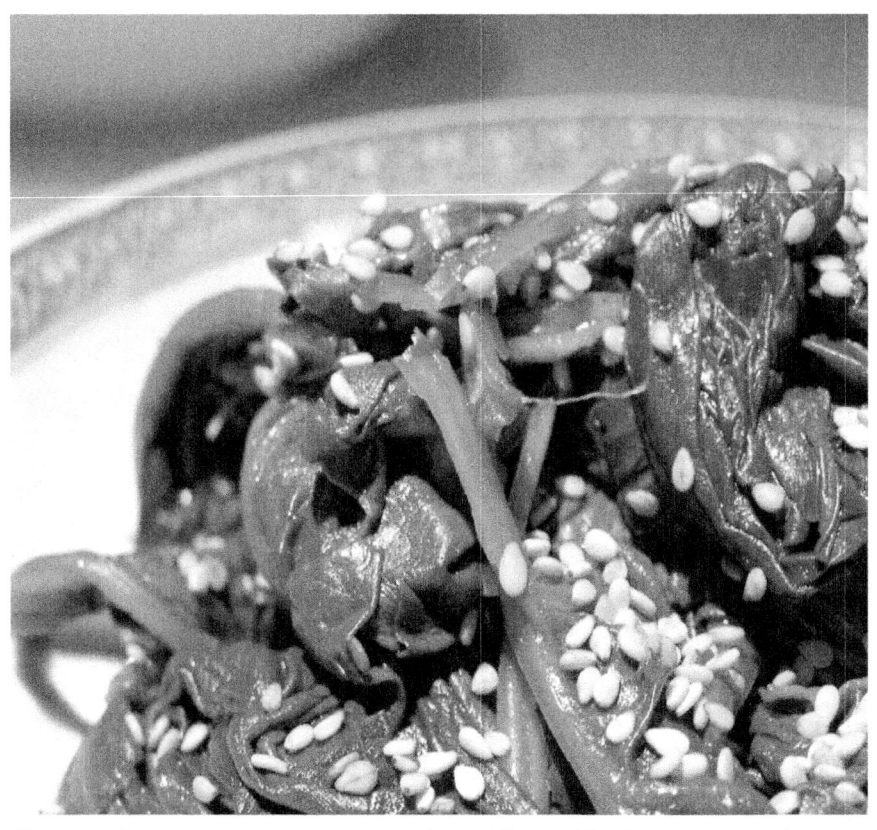

Here we have a super easy recipe that will quickly become your favorite snack.

Serves: 2

Time: 15 minutes

Ingredients:

- Spinach – 8 ounces
- Sesame oil – 1 ½ teaspoons
- Sesame seed – 2 teaspoons
- Soy sauce – 1 ½ teaspoons
- Green onion (chopped) – 1
- Garlic (minced) – 1 clove

Directions:

1. Set your spinach on in boiling water to blanch for about 30 seconds, remove and place in very cold water.

2. Let the spinach drained and squeeze out the excess water.

3. Mix the spinach with other ingredients including sesame oil, soy sauce, sesame seeds, minced garlic and green onion together.

4. Serve.

Kiwi and Mango Yogurt

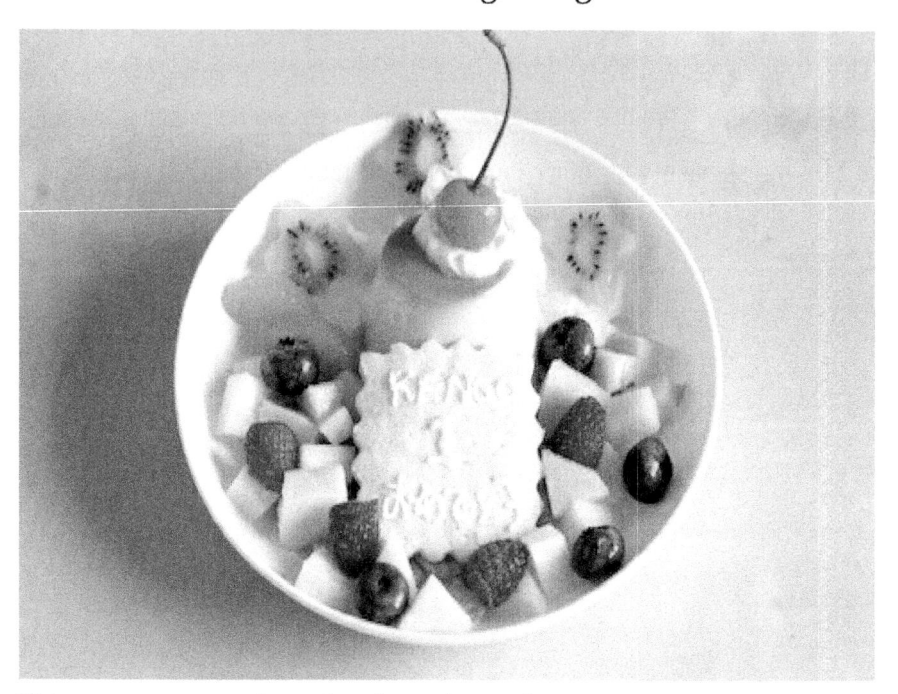

This tasty yogurt snack can be whipped up in five minutes or less.

Serves: 1

Time: 5 minutes

Ingredients:

- Kiwi (½-inch cubes) – ½ cup
- Mango (½ inch cubes) – ½ cup
- Yogurt – ½ cup

Directions:

1. Add all your ingredients in a bowl. Stir to combine.
2. Serve.

Kale and Spinach Smoothie

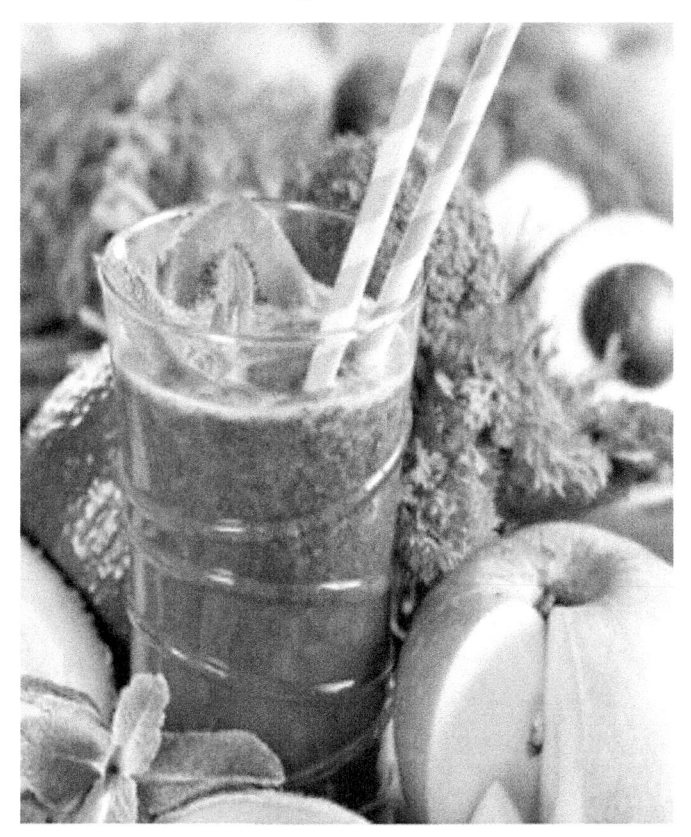

This delicious smoothie is the perfect way to start a long busy day.

Serves: 4

Time: 10 minutes

Ingredients:

- Kale – 1 cup
- Baby spinach – 1 cup
- Pineapple (diced) – 1 cup
- Banana – ½
- Cottage cheese – ½ cup
- Honey – 2 tablespoons
- Ice cube – 12 cubes

Directions:

1. Add all your ingredients in a blender. Process until smooth and combined.

2. Pour in a glass and serve.

Vietnamese Rice Noodle

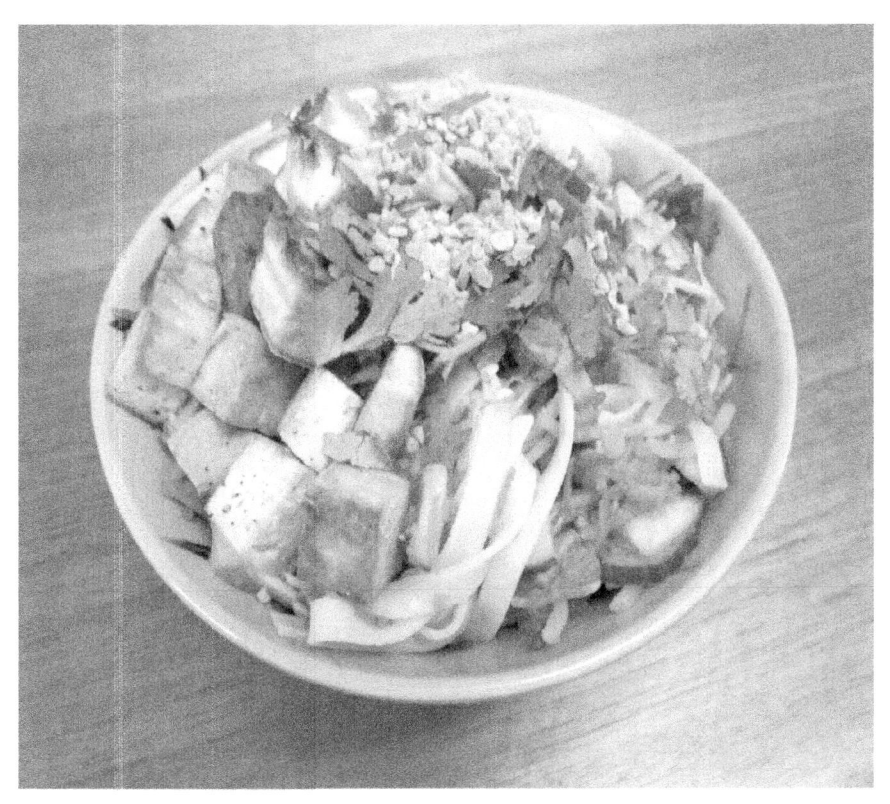

This noodle bowl is easy to make and super filling.

Serves: 4

Time: 30 minutes

Ingredients:

- Dried rice noodle – 12 ounces
- Cabbage leaves – 4
- Carrot (julienned) – 2
- Cucumber (thinly small and long slices) – 1
- Cilantro (chopped) – 1 cup
- Fish sauce – 3 tablespoons
- Garlic (minced) – 5 cloves
- Jalapeno pepper – ½ teaspoon

- Lime juice – ¼ cup
- Sugar – 3 tablespoons
- Unsalted peanut – ¼ cup
- Fresh mint (chopped) – 4 sprigs

Directions:

1. In a bowl, mix garlic, fish sauce, sugar, lime juice, cilantro and pepper together, stir well. Set aside.

2. Set your water over high heat to boil, season well with salt then add dried noodle for 3 minutes. Remove the noodle and place it to a container of cold water then drain it well. Let it cool.

3. Pour mixture of fish sauce to the noodle, add carrot, cucumber and cabbage, mix them well. Top with peanuts and mint.

4. Serve.

Spinach and Cheese Cups

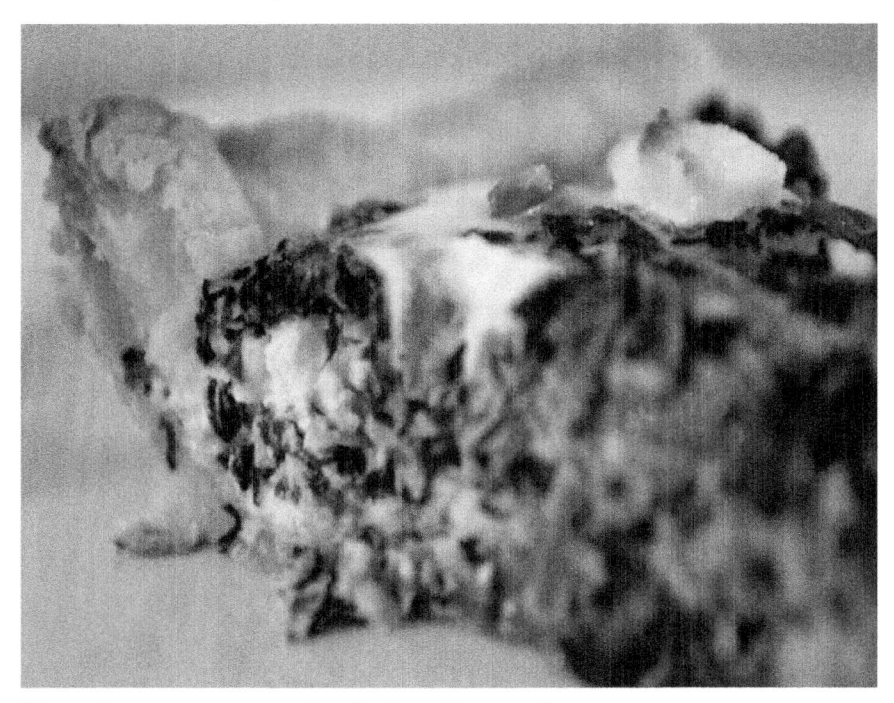

These cheese cups are perfect for breakfast on the go.

Serves: 3

Time: 25 minutes

Ingredients:

- Spinach (chopped) – 1 cup
- Shredded Cheddar Cheese – 1 cup
- Egg – 12
- Onion powder – 2 teaspoons
- Salt and pepper

Directions:

1. Preheat the oven to 400 degrees

2. Break eggs and place in a bowl then add cheese, chopped spinach, eggs and onion powder and season with salt and pepper.

3. Brush oil on the bottom of muffin tins then pour the mixture into them, about 12 cups. Cook for 10 minutes.

4. Remove and serve.

Baked Garlic Chicken

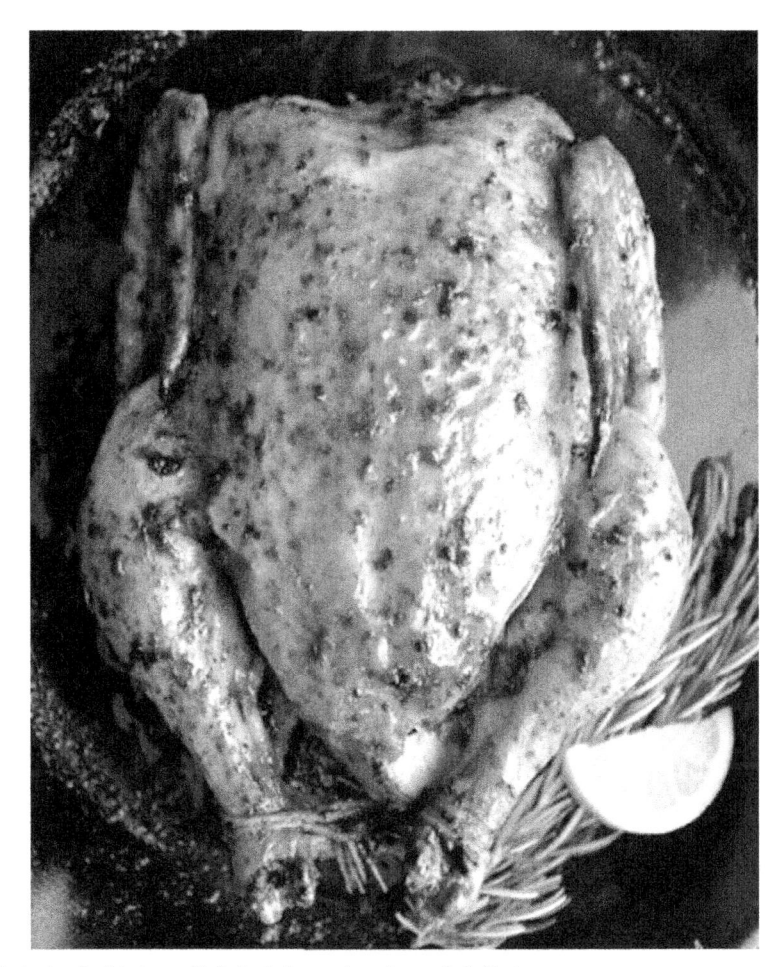

This baked chicken dish is juicy, simple and delicious.

Serves: 4

Time: 30 minutes

Ingredients:

- Chicken breast – 3 pounds (48 ounces)
- Grated Parmesan cheese – 12 tablespoons
- Olive oil – 4 tablespoons
- Breadcrumbs – 2/3 cup

- Chopped garlic – 5 cloves
- Garlic salt – ¼ teaspoon

Directions:

1. Preheat the oven to 425o F.

2. Let olive oil be heated in a pan, then add garlic and garlic salt to blend the flavor.

3. Mix the breadcrumbs and grated parmesan cheese together in a bowl.

4. Dip chicken breasts into the mixture of garlic and olive oil, then dip into the mixture of breadcrumbs and grated parmesan cheese, put all in baking dish.

5. Put the baking dish of chicken breasts in the oven and let it sit for 30 minutes, then serve.

Spinach and Kiwi Smoothie

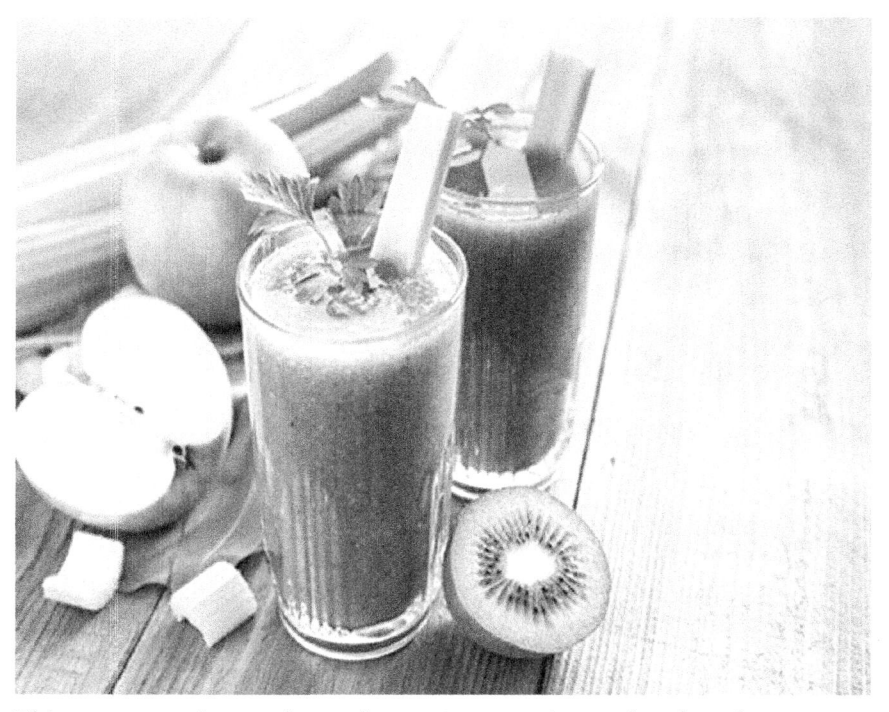

This tasty smoothie can be made in minutes and is perfect for a hot summer day.

Serves: 2

Time: 5 minutes

Ingredients:

- Baby spinach – 1 cup
- Kiwi (peeled) – 2
- Banana – ½
- Yogurt – ½ cup
- Ground flax seed – 2 tablespoons
- Apple juice – ½ cup
- Ice cube - 10

Directions:

1. Add all your ingredients in a blender. Process until smooth and combined.
2. When it's ready, pour it in 2 glasses and serve.

Asian Pineapple Chicken Stir Fry

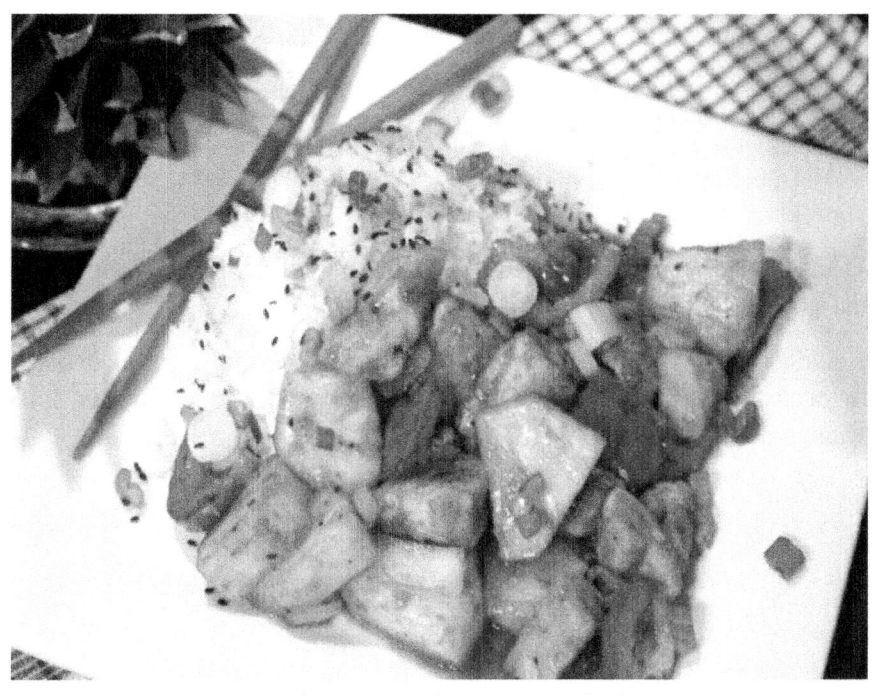

Pineapple is a delicious fruit enjoyed raw or cooked. This tasty recipe is perfect for the whole family.

Serves: 4

Time: 30 minutes

Ingredients:

- Chicken breast (skinless and boneless) – 1 pound
- Pineapple (cut into slices) – 1 cup
- Cornstarch – 2 tablespoons
- Ginger (chopped) – 1 teaspoon
- Cooking oil – 2 tablespoons
- Fish sauce – 1 tablespoon
- Garlic (minced) – 1 clove
- Thai Pineapple and chili sauce – ½ cup

Directions:

1. Mix cornstarch and fish sauce well together in a bowl, then place chicken in the mixture.

2. Set a tablespoon of oil on medium heat to get hot in a skillet on medium high heat and add garlic and ginger, stir fry for 30 seconds, then add pineapple, stir and cook for 3 minutes.

3. Add pineapple and Chile sauce, cook for 3 minutes more, then remove from skillet.

4. Add 1 tablespoon of oil to the same skillet, let it heat, then add the chicken and stir fry until chicken is cooked through, often for 5 minutes.

5. Add the cooked pineapple to the skillet, stir well together and cook until all are heated through, often 5 minutes more, then remove from heat, and it is better to pair with rice.

Raspberry, Strawberry and Blueberry Smoothie

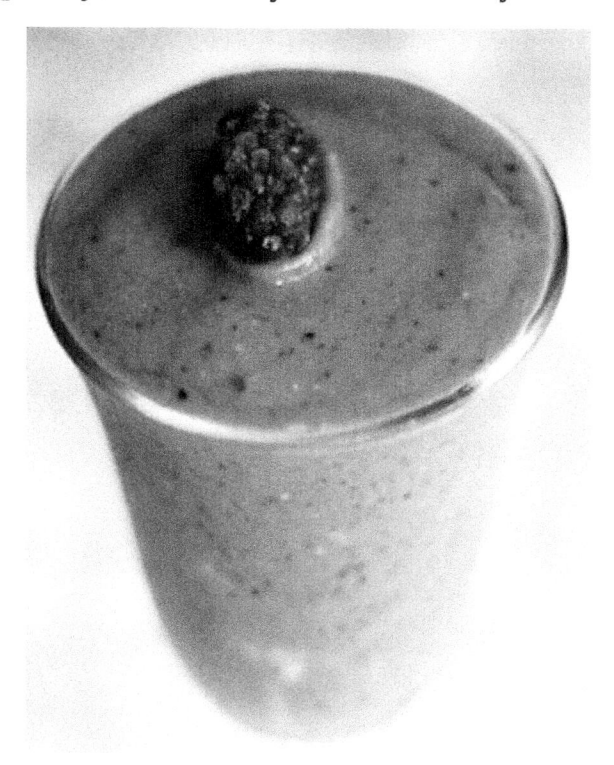

This mixed berry smoothie is naturally sweet, refreshing and tasty.

Serves: 3 - 4

Time: 10 minutes

Ingredients:

- Raspberry – 1 cup
- Strawberry – 1 cup
- Blueberry – ½ cup
- Water – ¼ cup
- Honey – 2 tablespoons
- Cottage cheese – ½ cup
- Ice cube – 12 cubes.

Directions:

1. Add all your ingredients in a blender. Process until smooth and combined.
2. Pour it in a glass and serve. Enjoy!

Pea Chicken Stir Fry

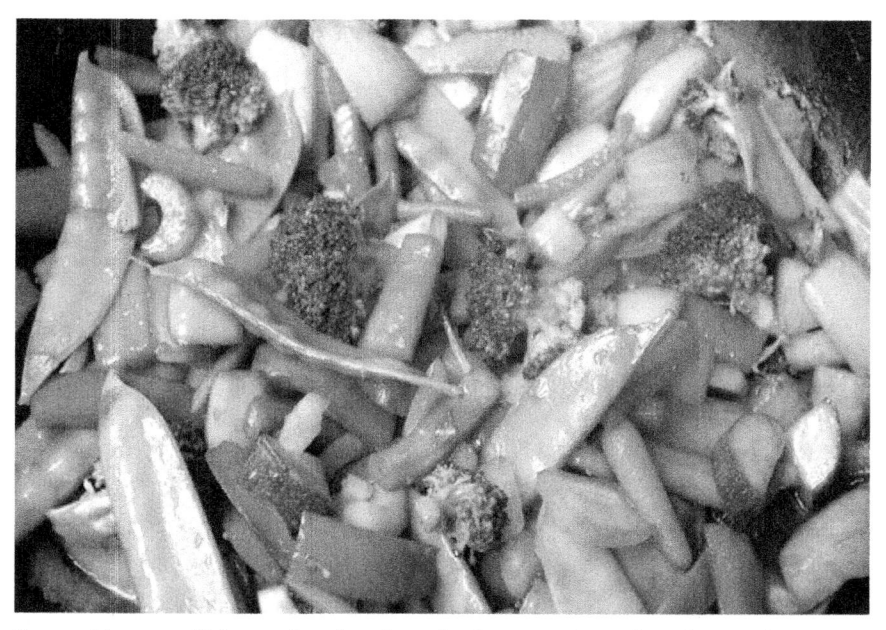

Serve this tasty dish as a late lunch or do three servings for a heavy dinner.

Serves: 2 - 3

Time: 30 minutes

Ingredients:

- Boneless chicken breasts (cut into strips) – 3 pounds
- Green bean – 4 ounces
- Soy sauce – 1 tablespoon
- Lemon juice – 3 tablespoons
- Honey – 1 teaspoon
- Black pepper – 1 teaspoon
- Green onion and lemon zest for garnish (optional)
- Olive oil – 2 tablespoons
- Garlic (chopped) – 2 cloves

Directions:

1. Let olive oil heated in a pan over medium heat.

2. Add garlic and cook for 2 minutes and add chicken to the pan, stir and cook for 5 minutes.

3. Add green beans to the pan, soy sauce, honey and lemon juice, stir well and cook for 7 minutes or until the beans are tender, then add black pepper.

4. Add green onion and adjust the season as desired and remove from heat.

5. Serve with rice.

Beet, Raspberry, Strawberry and Mango Smoothie

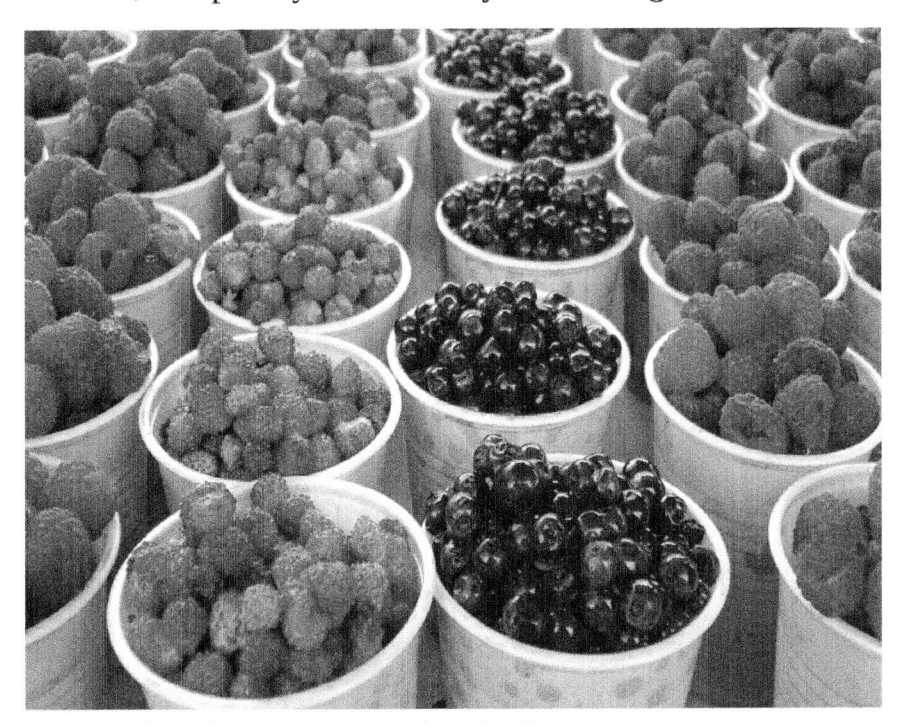

This smoothie is heathy, easy to make and delicious.

Serves: 4

Time: 15 minutes

Ingredients:

- Beet (peeled and shredded) – 1 cup
- Raspberry – 1 cup
- Strawberry (sliced) – 1 cup
- Mango (cut into chunks) – 1 cup
- Pineapple (cut into chunks) – 1 cup
- Avocado – 1
- Banana – 2
- Vanilla – 2 teaspoons

Directions:

1. Add all your ingredients in a blender. Process until smooth and combined.
2. When the mixture is smooth, pour in 4 glasses, then serve.

Miso Honey Chicken

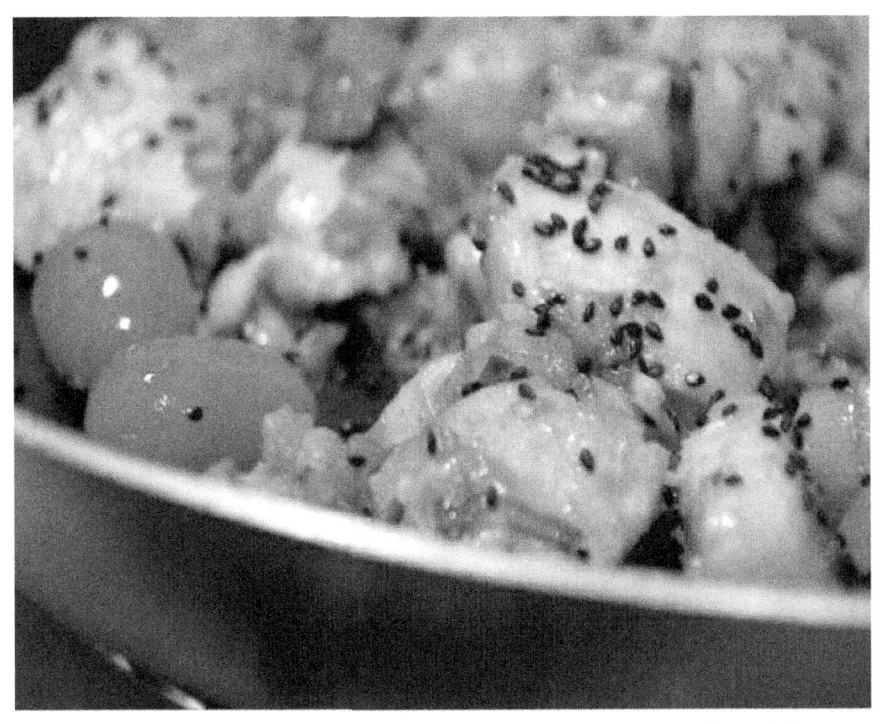

This juicy chicken plays on sweet and salty to create one succulent dish.

Serves: 4

Time: 15 minutes

Ingredients:

- Chicken breasts – 4 pounds
- Honey – ½ cup
- White miso paste – ½ cup
- Sesame oil – 3 teaspoons
- Crushed red pepper – ½ teaspoon

Directions:

1. Preheat the grill to the medium heat.

2. Add honey, sesame oil, miso pastes and crushed red pepper to a bowl, then mix them well together.

3. Brush over the top of chicken breasts with mixture of honey and sesame oil.

4. Grill the chicken breasts for 5 minutes for each side.

5. They're ready to serve.

Peach and Mango Smoothie

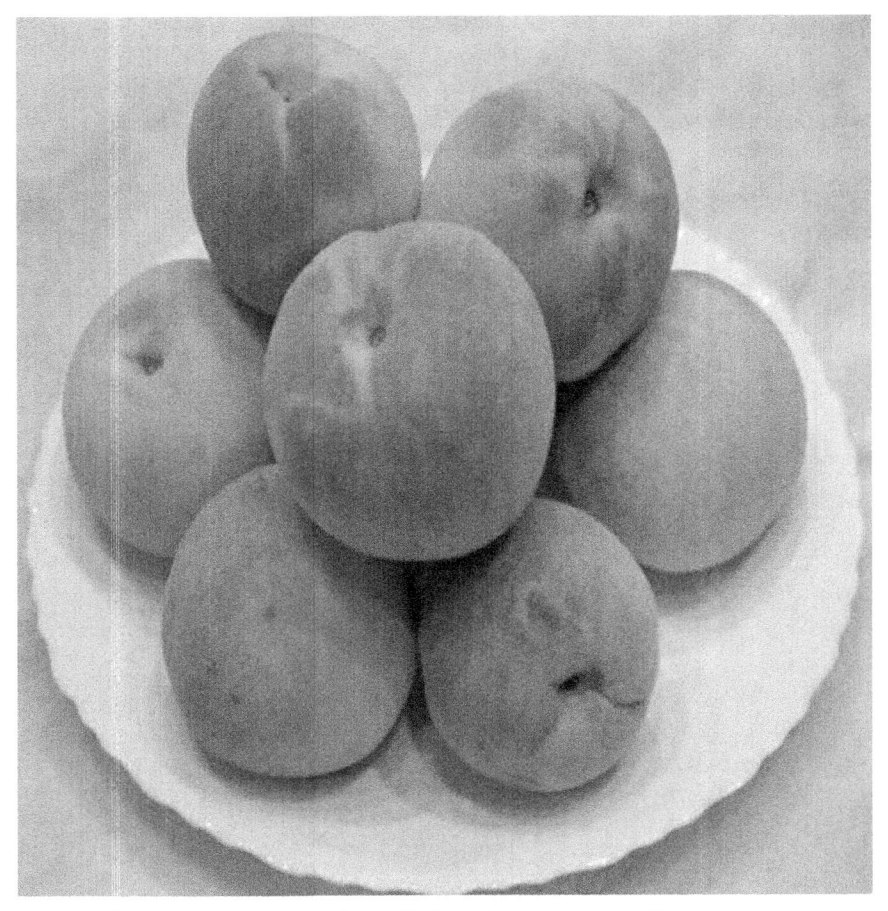

Here we have a tropical mix that will knock your boots off.

Serves: 2 - 3

Time: 10 minutes

Ingredients:

- Peach (diced) – 1 cup
- Mango (diced) – 1 cup
- Water – ¼ cup
- Cottage cheese – ½ cup
- Honey – 2 teaspoons

- Ice cube – 10 cubes

Directions:

1. Put all the ingredients including peach, mango, water, honey, cheese and ice cubes in a blender.

2. Mix them well until smooth.

3. Serve.

Simple and Quick Avocado Smoothie

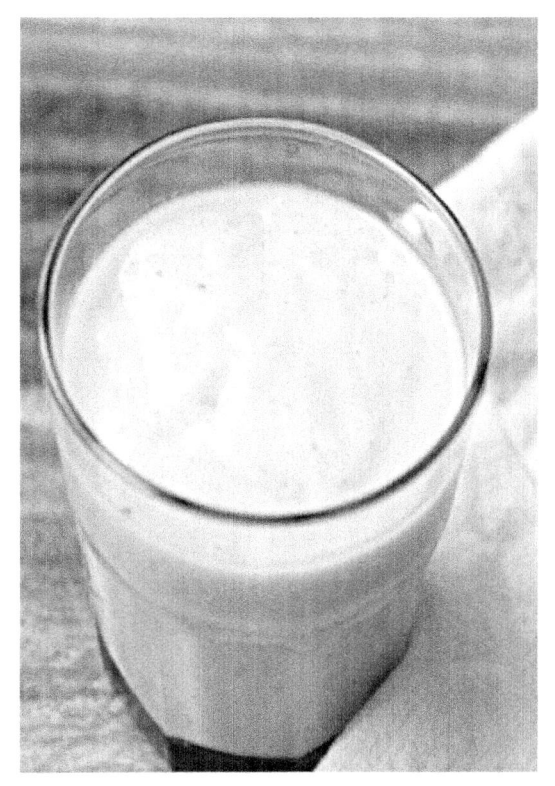

Try a glass of this creamy smoothie for a rich dose of healthy fat on any day of the week.

Serves: 1

Time: 7 minutes

Ingredients:

- Avocado (cut into cubes) - 2
- Milk – ½ cup
- Sugar – 2 tablespoons
- Ice cube – 4 cubes

Directions:

1. Add avocado, ice cubes, sugar and milk in a food processor.

2. Mix them well until smooth.

3. Pour the mixture in a glass and serve.

Minute Thai Chicken Stir Fry

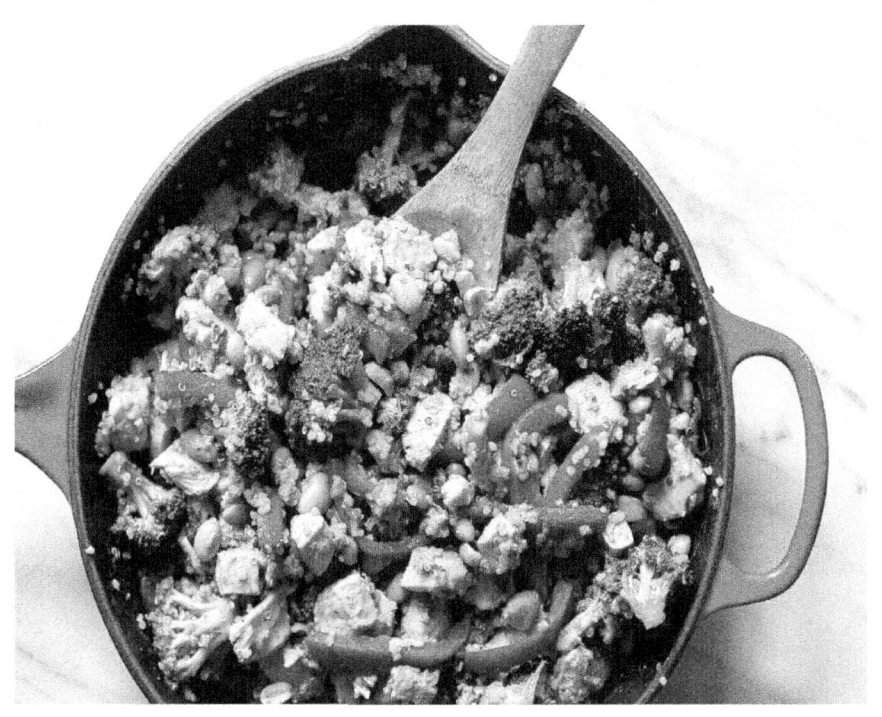

Here we have a 10 minute meal that makes a great dinner for two.

Serves: 2

Time: 10 minutes

Ingredients:

- Boneless chicken (cut into ¾ inch pieces) – 1 pound
- Cooking oil – 2 tablespoons
- Garlic (chopped) – 2 cloves
- Onion (thin slices) – ½ cup
- Fish sauce – 2 tablespoons
- Sugar – 2 tablespoons
- Thai Chile – 1 or more (optional)

Directions:

1. Set your oil over medium heat in a wok to get hot. Add garlic and stir for

30 seconds, when the garlic gets fragrant then add chicken, cook and stir for 5 minutes.

2. Add onion, fish sauce and Chile to the wok, and cook for 3 minutes more.

3. When the chicken is cooked through, taste it to adjust the season as desired then remove the wok from heat.

4. Then serve with rice.

Avocado Yogurt

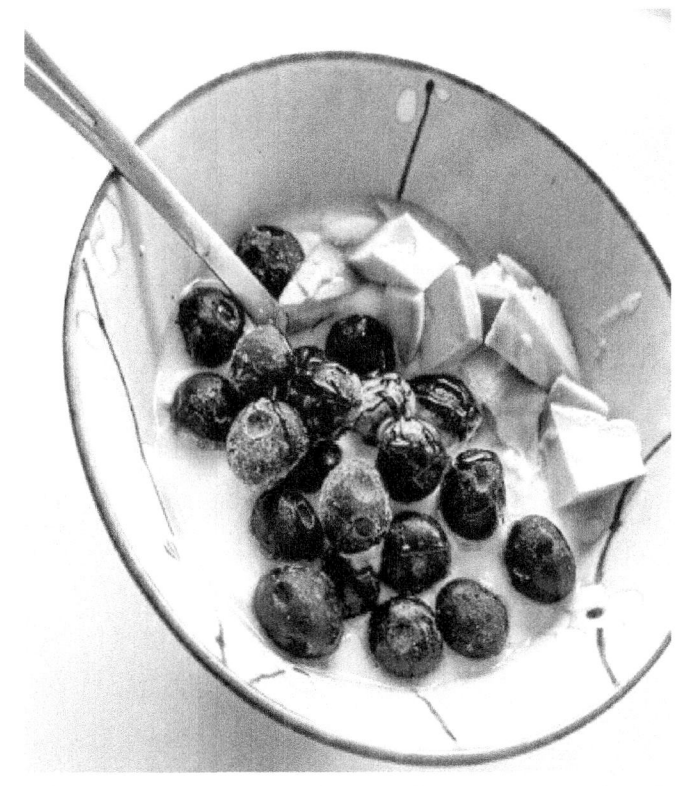

This avocado yogurt makes a quick tasty dip to be enjoyed with chips or crudites.

Serves: 1

Time: 5 minutes

Ingredients:

- Yogurt – ¼ cup
- Avocado (cut into cubes) – 1

Directions:

1. Pour the yogurt to avocado cubes in a glass or a bowl.

2. Serve.

Chicken Noodle and Ginger Sauce

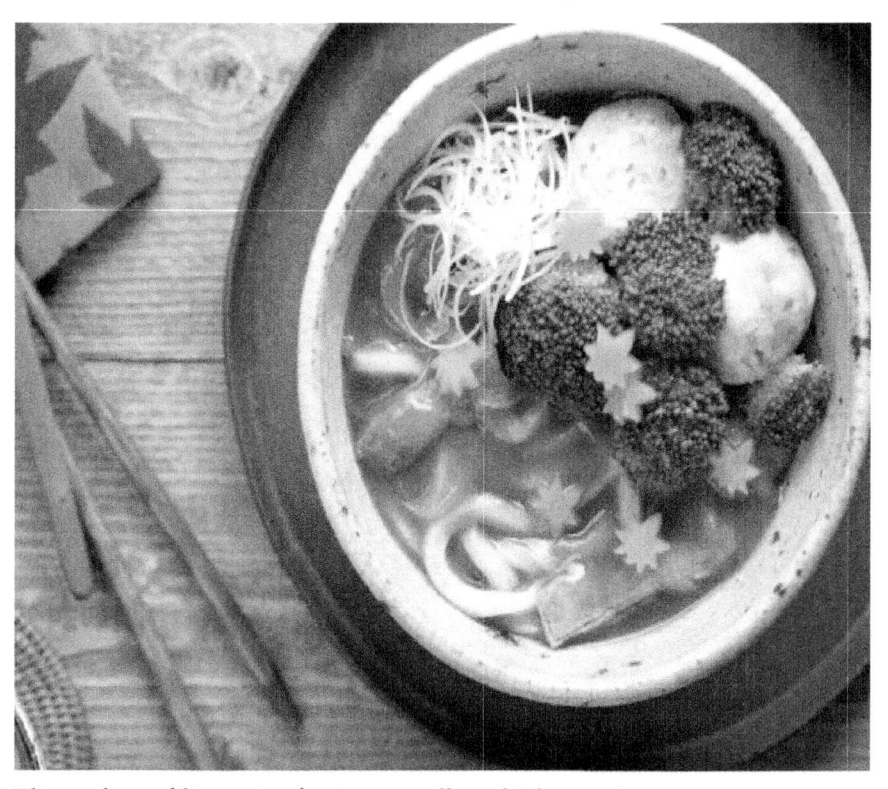

This makes a filing mix of spices, noodles, chicken and ginger.

Serves: 6

Time: 30 minutes

Ingredients:

- Cooked chicken – 3 cups
- Rice noodle – 6 ounces
- Carrot (cut into matchstick) – 2
- Red pepper (cut into small and long slices) – 1
- Roasted peanut (chopped) – ½ cup
- Water – 8 cups
- Vinegar – 2 tablespoons

For the sauce:

- Peanut butter – ½ cup
- Lime juice – 4 ½ tablespoons
- Soy sauce – 3 tablespoons
- Honey – 3 tablespoons
- Ginger (chopped) – 2 tablespoons
- Sesame oil – 1 ½ teaspoons
- Vinegar – 3 tablespoons
- Kosher salt – ¼ teaspoon
- Crushed chili – ¼ teaspoon

Directions:

1. Set your sauce ingredients on in your blender, then process until smooth.

2. Boil water in a pot, when it is boiled, often for 10 – 15 minutes, add vinegar and a bit of salt to the pot, add dried noodle and cook for 3 minutes.

3. Place noodle in a cold water, drain it well.

4. Pour the sauce into the noodle, add carrots and red pepper, mix them well, top with the peanuts.

5. Serve.

Conclusion

First of all. Congrats, on your beautiful bundle of joy. The food you eat from this point will greatly impact the health and livelihood of your growing fetus, and I am happy you gave me the opportunity to assist you with this aspect of your journey.

The foods you can actually enjoy during these months are a God send. So, I hope these 30 recipes will continue to serve as a delicious train of nutrition for your whole family.

Your review helps a lot so drop your feedback of these dishes on the platform you bought your book if you loved the meals you prepared. Until next time, have a safe delivery.

Printed in Great Britain
by Amazon